Table of Contents

A GUIDE FOR FASTING...

Great Healing!

Humanity has always been searching for new healing practices, remedies, therapies, medicines and miraculous discoveries for all the diseases we suffer.

The worst is that we keep getting new illnesses, and new viruses.

I'm not an authority in the field, I'm just a regular person, just like you, but out of my own experiences is that I have decided to write this guide.

My hope is that it may help people and probably even doctors on researching more about the most wonderful resource we all have in our bodies.

If at least this guide helps one person get cured after the person knows of the existence of a fatal illness, I will feel I have helped in opening a door to a new healthy future, and the writing of this guide would have been worth it.

September 24, 1997
Flagstaff, AZ

PREFACE

Many years ago, I started getting drawn to people who were vegetarians, macrobiotics, used alternative healing techniques, etc.

I do believe that our body is certainly the reflection of what we eat, and this is so important that not only it affects our physical body but our psyche as well.

If you look at different cultures throughout the world, and see what their most common diet is, you will be able to find some interesting facts, and I'm just going to name a few and let you think more about this...

In the Middle East, a lot of red meat is consumed; "raw meat" is very popular... People tend to be very passionate, explosive, temperamental, and conflictive....

In India, where cows are sacred, and meat is not so popular, people tend to be more focused, spiritual, peaceful...

Five years ago, I had the opportunity to lead a very different type of life. I was by the Amazon, in the southern region of Venezuela. My husband and I built a house ourselves. It had solar energy; we had our own natural water creek and pond. We didn't live with as much stress as we do here and now. The reason I'm telling you this, is because the circumstances were very favorable to start my experience.

I didn't have a schedule to meet, or any invoices to pay, so, that's when I was doing a lot of reading and a lot of work with the farm, we grew our own vegetables, had chickens, fruit trees, lots of house pets; dogs, cats, geese, etc.

I was living very close to Nature, and I could relate very well to all natural elements, one of the very first things you notice when you pay attention, is that when an animal gets sick, the very first thing it does, is to stop eating.

The animal will get a shady place to rest and drink a lot of water, most of the time they heal themselves by just doing so.

That is the natural best healing alternative we have, and it's no secret. A lot has been written about fasting, both for the physical therapeutically reasons, as for spiritual ones.

As late back as Hypocrites in the Fifth Century, he referred to fasting as to one of the best remedies for healing a sick body.

Back then, I had the opportunity to meet a lady who had been diagnosed with Leukemia, she had followed all traditional treatments but her situation just got worse. One day, after meeting a person who told her he could help her, she decided to fast. And she did, she was completely cured! No traces of anything after that. She is leading a very healthy life after 15 years. Meeting her, really impressed me, and just because of my curious nature, I started to search for books, people, find out about more experiences until the point where I decided to fast, and so I did during 16 days; I only drank water, preceded by three days of only juices. At the end of the water fast I only drank juices before I started eating, so that was a total of 21 days of liquids only. I kept a diary of all my experience. Then some friends of mine got enthusiastic about fasting, and this is what this guide is going to be about.

I used as main guide a wonderful book written by "Alexi Suvorin", a Russian publicist, who during the beginning of the Century did a lot of studies on fasting, and during a 4-year period he fasted for more than 200 days (approximately 50 days per year). He was monitored at a clinic in Belgrade during one of his 40 day fast, and there were medical proofs of his treatment. Alexi Suvorin helped more than 10 thousand people get cured from numerous diseases, many of them "incurable".

Unfortunately, nowadays, nobody has heard of him, and his studies have only been translated from Russian to Spanish and Arabic.

Medicine is a very profitable business, if it was going to be discovered that we all have the natural ways to heal, it would be quite dramatic for the whole "business".

On the other hand, there are many real doctors, who truly believe in natural ways of healing and in preventive medicine.

Now before concluding this preface, I must say what has really moved me into writing about fasting.

In the past four years I have lost three dear friends who died at a quite young age of cancer. The very first one who passed away, Michael had found out about his cancer and died within three months. Michael used to smoke two packs of cigarettes a day, he ate red meats in every single meal and would constantly make jokes like: "I'm a vegetarian in a second degree, a cow eats the grass and I eat the cow" I told him so many times about trying a fast, but he was a very stubborn person. The very last day I saw him alive, I gave him the book by Alexi Suvorin, and he finally promised to read it. Unfortunately he died three days later.

Then, Hilda, she was like a second mother to me. Ten years ago, the doctors diagnosed her with cancer. At that time, she went to chemotherapy but at the same time followed a natural treatment by an incredible doctor, Keshava Bhat. She healed and changed her eating habits and quit smoking.

After nine years, different circumstances made her start eating again all sort of meats, drink coffee and she started smoking again. Within four months, she was diagnosed with cancer again. I begged her to fast, she really wanted to do it, but didn't find an adequate place where to do it. She died a month later.

And finally, Margit, ironically she had been vegetarian for many years; had always taken care good care of herself, and died of cancer. In this particular case, probably a fast could have helped. But I also believe that there are certain situations in which nobody can do anything, when you're meant to go... that's it. But if you have a chance to try the best natural healing method and cure yourself, I'm sure it will be worth giving it a try.

Now, for the past three years, I have usually dreamt about offering a place where people can go to fast, and receive guidance and appropriate attention, for all important facets, getting into the fast, fasting and the most delicate phase: getting out of it.

This hasn't been easy to achieve, and last week, talking to a friend, he said; why don't you start writing about this? Actually I hadn't thought about it, but now I know I can soon have a guide that can help people, and then depending on the results, hopefully fasting centers could be created.

Please read this guide at least twice before you consider starting a fast, and ALWAYS get professional opinion and help.

Hope this guide will help you bring a bright healthy and rejuvenated new YOU!

WHAT IS A FAST?

There are a lot of ways for fasting, people use fruit juices, vegetable juices, a lot of people fast one day a week, others do it for three days once a month, and basically all these approaches are very good for maintaining a general well-being. But Fasting, really is only based on drinking water, all of the "Juice" fasts, are simply a mono-diet.

Most of you probably have only heard about a 40-day fast done by Jesus and you think this is just for very religious people, monks in the Tibet and great yogis.

Well, that's not the case, and in this guide I'm going to focus on fasts when you only take WATER.

A Fast consists in depriving your body from digesting foods, and giving it a chance to get rid of all toxins accumulated throughout your entire life. A fast must be VOLUNTARY (if it's not, the person may suffer a heart failure in two to three days), so when a fast is done at own will and it's complete, the stomach changes its function of digesting foods to a function of eliminating all kind of residues and toxins in our body, eliminating 95% of all known illness from its very root.

Once the body stops assimilating, it starts eliminating. A fast allows all the organs in your body to adopt a "slow motion function" and it balances, creating a balance of all energies and a re-birth of all cells in your body. It has a very rejuvenating effect, people comment out of their experiences the incredible look about their skin, "just like a baby's" it's a very common phrase.

A 40-day Fast can work miracles on a body. This should ONLY be done with the help of an expert or doctor.

A fast not only helps your physical body, but your mental and even spiritual realities.

The incredible discoveries of Alexis Suvorin were based that once the body starts fasting, the intestines adopt a quite passive role, and the elimination process instead of being expulsed through the intestines, start being expulsed through the saliva in the mouth.

That is why generally after 48 to 72 hours of fasting there's absolutely no appetite, there is a funny flavor constantly in the mouth, and if going through a long fast, the flavor and smell of your mouth is terrible. During a 40 day fast, the tongue goes through a very particular process: "During days 30 and 31 it gets a yellowish color in the center and like a white outline. During days 32, 33, right in the center of the tongue a brown spot appears. Days 34, 35, the spot grows bigger; the white outline starts disappearing, and the yellow stars diminishing. Days 35, 36, the yellow almost disappears, and the brown spot starts to reduce in size (at this time the last residues of the combustion produced in your body are getting out) Days 38,39, the tongue is almost red, just in the upper part there's a small yellow-brown circle, the end of residues in the "sewer" is coming out.

Day 40, the brownish spot disappears, the tongue has a healthy reddish overall, and for the first time during the fast, the person will feel hungry. The natural process lets you know your body is ready.

Under no circumstances anybody should keep on fasting after this has been completed, it may take 39 days with one person or 41 for another, but never more. If a person persists on fasting, it will be a voluntary suicide.*

The fast process is as perfect and natural as a woman needs 9 months to bring a child into this world. Once the profound cleansing has been achieved, your body will let you know.

One of the most dangerous steps in fasting is getting out of the fast, and I will dedicate lots of attention to this further on.

In general, 5, 10 to 15 days of fasting are very beneficial, and essential to prepare yourself for a complete cleansing of 40 days. Just with a fatal illness, when there's not much time left, a person should try to go all at once for the 40 day fast, and ALWAYS under supervision of a doctor or expert.

Don't think that fasting is 100% effective for ALL circumstances, but it is 95% for most of them, and depending on the condition of the individual, I think you ought to give it a try. If somebody is dying, knows that has a couple of months left, has to be under strict therapies and drugs, why not give the body a natural resource for healing itself. If the person does not make it, at least the very last days will be without all the painful surrounding, medicine, drugs. And you know the person may have a big chance of healing. Otherwise, death will be imminent also, and cost you a lot of pain, no HOPE, and a fortune.

I hope that soon we will all be able to look back, and see these days as primitive ones. Today most people and doctor's say: "the patient is very ill, let's feed him, so he can gain all his energy back", and will feed the person sometimes against his will with a glass of milk, hot chicken or beef soup, too much protein!!

The best of Nature is its simplicity; simple facts characterize real truth and virtue.
Animals fast, even Nature rests in winter, and then the beauty of new sprouts comes out in spring. There are no hidden secrets in all of this, we just have to open our eyes and see...

* "Healing through Fasting", Alexi Suvorin.

WHO CAN FAST? ...

How does a Fast affect your Body?

Fasting is not recommended for children. Their bodies are developing so just in some extreme cases of disease a fast could be done to help them heal. Alexi Suvorin tells in his writings about several children with diabetes who got cured with short period fasts 3 to 6 days, which were repeated constantly until the sugar in the blood completely disappeared. This short term fasts will definitely help children heal, but never a child should do a long term fast.

Suvorin also talks about very many cases of people in their 60's and 70's doing 40 day fasts, which cured them of a whole variety of diseases, in many cases diseases that people had throughout their lives.

Basically it is important to note that in order to heal through a fast, any person, no matter how weak may be, has the physical strength needed, it really all depends on their psychic strength and will of power to go through a fast, that's all it takes.

Alexi Suvorin, Dr. Roux and Dr. Guelpa explain about the fasting process:
"The life of a red cell is of 6 weeks, a 40 day fast takes also 6 weeks, so then you would say, what a horrifying story, by the end of the fast I would have no blood! but that's not the way it happens.

During a fast, the body keeps producing 80% of the normal amounts of blood, and since your body perceives a change in its routine, it reacts to it, the same way as white cells increase in production when they sense the threat of a disease.

Since we are not providing any food, the body looks for what is available, so it first takes all the sick and weak cells of the blood, later it takes all the unnecessary accumulated salts and toxins, next the calcified residues which normally never gets expulsed from our bodies and is the main cause of SCLEROSIS.

subsequently it takes the iron of bad quality that had been deposited in the liver, it also takes the accumulated fat, the sugar in the blood. Finally, our bodies, free from all that toxic baggage, start producing new red cells, even though they are going to be less in quantity, they are going to have a superior quality.

This explains how people with anemia and diabetes get cured. They also talked about the heart, they say a weak heart gets stronger in the very first days of a fast, being the heart one of the deposits of fat; once it is eliminated, the worn out muscles get more elasticity and new strength".

WHAT CAN A FAST CURE?

Do healthy people need to fast?

A Fast doesn't only have the properties of healing, but of purification and renewal of all cells, and more purification will take place in a healthier body. A healthy person will benefit after a fast, with new skin and muscles, a flush in the cheeks, a bright shine in the eyes, lots of energy, better concentration, etc.

A person fasting three to five continued days on a monthly basis would be able to see great results at the end of a year. During each fast, old skin is lost; it is substituted by rejuvenated skin. This can result in a marvelous rejuvenating process.

The short continued fasts, is what is most recommend for people who want to be cured from minor diseases, people who wish to be healthier, more vigorous and feel & look younger.

If proper exercise and eating habits are followed after each fast, the muscle strength can increase approximately 10 to 15%, just think what this could mean after four to five years.

Suvorin mentions about numerous diseases being healed. Among those he cites ulcers, anemia, diabetes, cancer, arteriosclerosis, asthma, emphysema, appendicitis, heart weakness, liver diseases, kidney stone, indigestion, constipation, neurosis, infections, rheumatism, skin disorders, sexually transmitted like syphilis, etc.

Among those 10.000 people that Suvorin guided, there were reports of a woman who had a severe case of periodontal disease, and all the gums got cured. There was a 72-year-old man, who got rid of age spots in his hands, his hair stopped falling, and started growing hair!

A lot of people reported a better sense of being, much more energy and great concentration.

FASTING.... People Experiences

I read a footnote on Suvorin's book, which refers to a Doctor here in the United States, back in the late 1800's, his name was Tanner. When he was 47 years old, he was terminally ill. It was a hopeless case. Being a doctor and believing in fasting, he got in a clinic and under very strict supervision, he did a 40 day fast. The very first days were a nightmare, the doctors in the clinic wouldn't let him drink water, get out of the room and the air wasn't fresh, it got a fetid odor. They wouldn't let him rest while sleeping, since everybody thought he could cheat at night, so they placed a big light on him. Finally after 14 days, they would let him take two walks a day, and he was able to drink water from a park fountain and breathe fresh air.

His fast started on June 28, 1880 and ended on August 7, 40 days. He healed, and broke his fast eating a peach, after that, he ate only melons, until he recuperated the 45 pounds he had lost. Dr. Tanner lived in very good health until nearly 90 years old. He helped a lot of his patients with fasting techniques.

Alexi Suvorin in Russia used to do short fasts regularly, he practiced three complete fasts of 40 days.

In Argentina, Monseñor Miguel Jaluf, back in 1930 worked on the translation of Suvorin's experiences, and he practiced a couple of fasts.

I have read about a lot of experiences, teachings and techniques in books by Hooker Dewey, Greg Brodsky, Yogi Ramacharaka, Petra Hopfenzitz and Doctor Hellmut Lutzner.

For the short fast periods you can do it by yourself at home, but for the purification fasts you need help and supervision. Hopefully find a clinic or center where you can fast while being monitored.

In Europe, these centers are more popular than in the States, especially in Germany.

A GOLDEN RULE

A MUST when fasting, is to practice daily water enemas, this is a very important step.

The intestines are passive and cannot dry; water lubricates them. But the most important aspect is that throughout your whole life a lot of toxins and deposits have been adhering to the walls of your duodenum, all those accumulated toxins, are the number one reason for most diseases.

You are not going to believe all kind of filth that comes out, even after many days of not feeding your body.

Seeing this, is what really gives you the strength to keep going on. You actually get to see what your body is getting rid off, even though the worst comes out through your saliva.

I have heard of many people applying laxatives and coffee enemas. I don't advise you to do this. You should allow your body to eliminate in a natural way, when you practice enemas, your body absorbs water and you don't want it to absorb such a toxic stimulant as coffee in that process.

If applying enemas in the appropriate way, you won't suffer from headaches in the fasting process. I repeat again, this is one of the most important steps along the way.

It is very important that in the 7-day preparation before going to a 40-day fast, you apply daily enemas and start getting comfortable about applying them. Later on, I will explain in detail how to do an effective enema.

HOW DID I START MY FAST?

First of all, I was totally determined to fast, I wanted to try a 14 day fast as a preparation to go into my 40 day fast.

There was nothing major wrong with me, well at least not that I knew about. The only incident had been that two weeks prior to my fast, I had visit my gynecologist for a regular exam, and he saw some white spots which he didn't like at all, he wanted to have them analyzed. I told him what I was about to do, and he practically quoted me as "crazy".

The reason for fasting was to experience a general deep cleansing. It was in 1992, as I told you before, I was in a very appropriate place. Besides taking care of the house and little farm, we had a small kiosk where we sold food and had a camping place. So my days were basically filled with food preparation.

As I was getting excited about fasting, I didn't want to keep on cooking on a daily basis, even though I had read about many people who kept on doing their daily activities.

I found a small cabin by a water creek in the jungle. It seemed to be the perfect place, and it was 20 minutes away from my home.

I took with me one of my dogs, Gypsie, a very lovable female German Shepherd who made me great company (of course she didn't fast!)

I equipped myself with a radio in order to keep in contact with my husband; there were no telephone lines down there, much less cellular phones. I also took a portable tape recorder in order to record my experience, a notebook, a lot of books and materials for making handcrafts.

I used to smoke a pack of cigarettes per day and drank a lot of coffee, so during the week of preparation I quit the coffee, started smoking less and I smoked my last cigarette the last day before the water fast. During the week of preparation you are not supposed to eat any meats or dairy products.

For the period of the seven days of preparation it is advisable to do the following:

First two days eat just fruits, vegetables, light grains like oatmeal and barley.

The following two days drop the grains and eat only vegetables (raw or cooked) and eat fruits or drink fruit juices.

The last three days, only drink fruit and vegetable juices.

During those seven days you must also drink as much water as possible.

That week, I was trying the enemas for the first time in my life, and I became so frustrated; I thought I was never going to be able to master the art.

I had a very strong desire to fast, I only felt hungry during the last three days of the preparation process while I was drinking juices. It was much more difficult for me to handle the cigarette cravings than the hunger.

I went to the cabin the last day of my preparation week. I remember it was a beautiful afternoon. Once I arrived, I arranged my belongings and made myself comfortable. Then I went out for a walk, went to the creek and checked all the surroundings. It was so exciting to be able to finally start!

The following morning my water fast began, it was November 10, 1992

MY DAILY EXPERIENCE FASTING

The first thing I did that morning was to weight myself and take my body temperature.

Some people like to take different measurements of different parts of their bodies to see how many inches they lose at the end, but I didn't do it. My concern wasn't about losing weight.

Then I had a glass of hot water. I went out and sat down to be able to receive the early sun in my body, that's very important, your body gets vitamins A & D. Then I took a walk of approximately two miles and got in the pond, where I stayed for long periods of time, imagining how my body was cleansing.

The sunbathing, morning walk and bath became a daily routine for me. Sometimes I would double or triple the walking distance. I never felt tired. On the contrary, there were mornings that I felt totally energized.

If I felt an urge or desire of getting something in my stomach I drank water, all the time it was room temperature, it is not advisable to drink iced water. The glass of hot water in the mornings is very good; it should be as hot as your body can take it comfortably.

In the afternoons I would read, take a nap, do some very light exercises outside and took another immersion bath in the pond and moved to the running water at the creek, which had quite a strong current, that felt great!

I started working on arts and crafts, I made quite a few adornments.

That first night I wrote in a piece of paper all the reasons why I wanted to fast and quit smoking and placed them in a visible place, so I could read them every time I needed reinforcement. I didn't feel hunger, just that smoking habit kept reminding me of how much I was missing it.

The urge for cigarettes was over by the end of the second day. On the second day, something happened to me. In the afternoon while walking to the river, I was wearing sandals. I left my sandals and clothing on the ground and went for my bath. Afterwards, when ready to go back to the cabin, I put on my sandal and I felt this horrible sting, it was very painful. I tried to see what had caused it, but didn't find anything.

Back in the cabin, I took my sandal off and found a huge black ant grasped to it. When I saw it, I recognized it, it has a popular name in the region "Veinticuatro" translates to "Twenty-four", this ant injects venom when it bites. It is known for giving 24 hours of high fever and causing much pain.

I did not get worried, I had taken with me a suction cup just in case, because in that area there are plenty of spiders, snakes, wasps and bees. Anyway, I didn't use the suction cup; I knew my body could only eliminate the venom. Earlier in my life, I had been bitten by a black scorpion, many wasps and bees. I knew how my body responded. Under normal circumstances, the pain would have been awful, the skin would have turned greenish and violet at the sting, and then a wider yellowish ring would have surrounded the area. This would have lasted three to seven days, been swollen and painful. That night, my foot got huge, very swollen and kind of purple, it was very itchy. The next morning, it was over! I couldn't believe it!

It was during my third day of fasting that I finally practiced an enema that really worked, I couldn't believe what came out. But the most incredible part is that from day 3 to 15, after my body had not received any food, all this filth kept coming out. It had the worst appearance, from substances that looked like white worms to very solid and hard black balls in the last days. The smell was unbearable!

During the seventh day of my fast, I got my period, I normally get some slight pain or discomfort. During the fast, I got almost no discomfort. The first three days were normal, then on the fourth day it stopped, and the following day, I started having this blackish fluid, it was very dark and had a strong smell, it lasted for eight days..! It must have taken out whatever I had, because the next time I went to the doctor, those white spots were gone.

During the twelve day, I took a very long walk of approximately eight miles; I didn't feel tired, I suppose all that exercise helped me, since that afternoon when I did my enema, a whole sewer came out..! Awful! Twelve days of water plus three previous days of juices, no solids, and all of that was still inside of me, it was hard to believe. This will definitely be one of the most striking aspects of the experience if you decide to fast.

My body temperature was steady throughout the whole fast, between 97 and 98,

I never felt fatigue, heavy drowsiness, did not suffer from vomits or headaches.

During the second week, the aspect of the saliva was getting very thick and sticky, the taste of it was getting worse every time, that is why everybody says that towards the 30th day you don't feel any appetite, and you can bet on it! It certainly becomes a sewer.

Please know that you NEVER CAN SWALOW your own saliva; you must have a recipient near you in order to be spitting all the time.

I noticed through the 16 days of water, that my hair and nails grew normally. During the first ten days I got a remarkable strength of my nervous system, but I was extremely sensible to noises, even as subtle as the wind, a bird singing..

I did urinate very frequently on a daily basis.

The most difficult thing for me to deal with was time. Days never seemed to end, I would start an activity, and thought that probably three hours had gone by, and eventually it had only been a half an hour.

Now, if you see how much time we dedicate to food every single day, thinking of what we are going to eat, preparing the food, preparing the table, cleaning afterwards or buying prepared food. This takes place three times a day, and sometimes, a lot of people as soon as they have nothing to do, will go for a snack. All of a sudden, when you don't have to worry for food, it's like you have all the time in the world.

Especially for me, at that time, when for more than a year, most of my time was dedicated to cooking for the kiosk, shopping and cleaning. Besides, I have been a person who cooks; I don't like ready meals that you just place in a microwave. So, a little detail like that was one of the most difficult things to deal with, I had much time available!

At the end of my fast, I was very sensitive; a nice song would make me cry. I broke my fast with a drop of honey on my tongue, then later when I had a glass of orange juice, the feeling was so extraordinary, I felt so thankful for the orange taste in my mouth, it was heaven, and I cried of happiness!

My handwriting that just before the fast had gotten to look as a doctor's became very eligible, uniform, small and beautiful!

My first two days after the fast I only took juices, on the third day I incorporated soups and purees, on the fifth day I incorporated grains. The only problem I suffered on the third day after solid food was that my foot got very swollen and that was because I ate big portions and should have eaten half of what I did.

If you eat too much quantity, your heart has to overwork to do the digesting process! That is why it is so delicate to go back to eating.

I lost 15 pounds; it wasn't that bad, the first days it was like I had a terrible flu, after a week and a half I was totally re-established and with an ideal weight.

There were radical changes in my life after the fast, and I couldn't find again the right moment to do the 40 day fast.

A lot of my friends got excited about my experience. And within two months, one of them, Harry, started a fast, he fasted during 29 days without stopping his work and he was feeling great. Harry was over 50 years old, I saw him one month after he had finished his fast and he looked great, not only that, he got a lot of vitality, which he pretty much needs since he is a tour guide and needs to walk miles and miles per day, ride boats, etc.

Then another friend, Victoria, decided to fast, she did it for 15 days and felt great too, she was 21 years old.

Since then, I met three people who had done a 40 day fast and cured themselves from the illnesses they were suffering. The only thing different in their fast, is that the water they took, was water where they had used for boiling a whole potato, yucca or a carrot. They said they weren't too sure about the minerals in the natural water. The only thing I did once in a while was to add a drop of lime juice to the hot water in the morning. Today if I had to do a long fast again, I would certainly omit the drop of lime, now I know the best is PURE water.

I have heard about the water quality at Mt. Shasta in California. They say it has no impurities and that it has a lot of minerals, I assume that it could be excellent water for doing a fast. If you are going to use bottled water, I recommend you re-energize the water before drinking it. You can do that by pouring a glass of water to an empty glass and back to the previous glass, do that several times. You will see the oxygen getting activated, that is very good.

HEALING BEYOND YOUR PHYSICAL BODY

While fasting, you will be able to see "through", it's like all of a sudden facing the REAL YOU. That is why we hear about so many fasting techniques among religious practices.

The mental clarity you get is astonishing; you start seeing your reality as it is.
This is why it is very important that the person fasting is not alone through the process.

You may have heard of shamanism techniques, where a shaman must go through several days of fasting and go all by himself to experience encounters with eagles, bears, etc. You have also heard about religious fasts, all of them helping the individual to get the clarity, inner peace and strength they are searching.

What happens is that you may experience an encounter with your higher self, you see clearly through your deepest levels. If you are not prepared for this stage, and you still hold a lot of fears and traumas in your life, the experience could be somehow scary.

If you are ready to face the facts, it may become one of the most beautiful and transcendental experiences of your life.

That is why I think, it would be ideal to find a place where there are several people fasting under supervision.

Where there are group activities for everybody to share, such as painting, even if you have not ever taken a brush in your hands before, listening to music, writing, handcrafts, reading poetry, watching movies that lift the spirit, a beautiful thing to do is to plant seeds, take care of the seedlings and watch them grow as the new you grows as well (never use chemicals for the plants while you are fasting, even the smell can be hazardous to your health).

It is very nice to read, try selecting books that are not controversial, but that lift the spirit and may be discussed in groups.

When fasting; you must keep active, you are not to remain in bed all day long. On the contrary, you should get up early in the morning and go to a place where you can receive the warmth of the early sun (not after 10 am), then you should walk a couple of miles at a comfortably slow rhythm, more than exercising it should be a walk where you are able to enjoy your surroundings, and obviously this cannot be done in downtown New York where you will be breathing carbon monoxide instead of clean air.

Taking immerse baths are highly recommendable, ideally at rivers, ocean or ponds, if they are going to be in swimming pools watch for the contents of chemicals in the water. You should take at least two baths a day. Then you can concentrate in different activities as the ones mentioned before. You may also want to keep a diary.

You could practice your daily enema in the morning or mid-afternoon, so then you can take another short walk, a bath end enjoy again the warm sunrays in the afternoon after 4 pm.

Fasting can be a great experience, depriving yourself from food only to gain new insights and a healthier you.

You get to appreciate life in a fuller way, you become aware of the simplest things, yet the grandest of them all... the singing of a bird, the aroma of a flower, shapes of clouds, the rainbow in a drop of water, the beauty and greatness of Nature, of God, the beauty in all of us!

You may see how simple everything really is, and how complicated we keep trying on making it.

When coming out of the fast, at that delicate stage is when you should never be alone and really watch how you incorporate food again to your diet. Once again, this is the most delicate phase. Not only with food, but also, if you are going to be thrown back to the hectic pace this world lives in all at once, your nervous system may not take it too well.

I absolutely recommend that while fasting and for the two or three weeks following a 40 day fast, you watch no television, don't listen to the radio and forget your daily "problems", you are going to be highly sensitive, so if there's a way to put everything on hold, do it.

After your fast, you may decide to keep a healthier diet, especially after seeing all the filth that came out, it may be just natural that you are really going to watch what you feed your body. Also you may decide to keep applying water enemas on a steady basis, if you decide to do so, once a week or bi-weekly may be one of the healthiest things you can keep on doing.

HOW TO APPLY A WATER ENEMA

The water temperature should be between 99 and 100 degrees. The best posture is to be lying down on your stomach or on your side.

You should place the container just above your body, not too high because the water could come out with high pressure and is not advisable.

Relax and breath deeply, try to get in as much water as possible. It is very difficult to achieve, but ideally, you should then stand-up, and very delicately massage your abdomen for some time. Then let everything out.

A good enema should take 20 to 45 minutes. Don't get frustrated if the first time you are not able to keep the water in for more than three minutes.

You should be very patient and persistent and then you will be able to apply them like an expert, and once you see how effective they are, you will want to practice them regularly.

A FINAL REMINDER

In writing this guide, I once again, wish to emphasize that I don't recommend anybody to practice fasting techniques without help from a doctor or expert.

I just wish to share with you some of my own experiences and knowledge from reading and meeting other people who have practiced fasts. I'm no doctor or expert, just a human being who feels there are other alternatives, and who has discovered the wonders of the marvelous design in our bodies, the miracle of creation in all of nature and us.

Coming out of the fast is very delicate. Eat very tiny portions, increment sizes very slowly. Reintroduce vegetable juices, purees and vegetarian soups. Slowly reintroduce grains like oatmeal and barley. Do not eat any meats or dairy products for the first week.

Please watch portions! Small tiny portions, if not, you may overwork your heart.

Keep drinking as much water as possible.

I wish you the best; hope you have lots of will power and a great experience.

Most Sincerely,

Mer Homei

www.ingramcontent.com/pod-product-compliance
Lightning Source LLC
Chambersburg PA
CBHW050922290526
45792CB00002B/851